Hallucino Truth Hallucinogenic Plants

The Ultimate Beginner's Guide to LSD, Peyote, Psilocybin, and PCP

Copyright 2015 by Colin Willis - All rights reserved.

This document is geared towards providing exact and reliable information in regards to the topic and issue covered. The publication is sold with the idea that the publisher is not required to render accounting, officially permitted, or otherwise, qualified services. If advice is necessary, legal or professional, a practiced individual in the profession should be ordered.

In no way is it legal to reproduce, duplicate, or transmit any part of this document in either electronic means or in printed format. Recording of this publication is strictly prohibited and any storage of this document is not allowed unless with written permission from the publisher. All rights reserved.

The information provided herein is stated to be truthful and consistent, in that any liability, in terms of inattention or otherwise, by any usage or abuse of any policies, processes, or directions contained within is the solitary and utter responsibility of the recipient reader. Under no circumstances will any legal responsibility or blame be held against the publisher for any reparation, damages, or monetary loss due to the information herein, either directly or indirectly.

The information herein is offered for informational purposes solely and is universal as so. The presentation of the information is without contract or any type of guarantee assurance.

The trademarks that are used are without any consent, and the publication of the trademark is without permission or backing by the trademark owner. All trademarks and brands within this book are for clarifying purposes only and are owned by the owners themselves, not affiliated with this document.

Table Of Contents

Introduction

Chapter 1: Brief Background of Hallucinogens

Chapter 2: Modern Developments

Chapter 3: Overview of LSD, Peyote, Psilocybin and PCP

Chapter 4: Pros and Cons

Chapter 5: Hallucinogens vs. Other Drugs

Conclusion

Introduction

You've probably heard of "Hallucinogens" at some point. Maybe you've heard about how they are supposed to give people who use them some semblance of euphoria and how they can somehow alter one's way of thinking. So, what exactly are hallucinogens and hallucinogenic plants?

Well, in this short and concise book, we will get into the various types of hallucinogens, the history of them, the science behind them, and how they can affect one's body. More practically, we will also look at the pros and cons of these substances and how they compare to each other.

In this book we are aiming to look at this topic in an unbiased light. We are not promoting the consumption of hallucinogens, per se, but we want to make sure that if someone is interested in this controversial topic, he or she can reach more informed conclusions.

We hope that you are able to learn a thing or two!

Chapter 1:

Brief Background Of Hallucinogens

What are they?

Hallucinogens are psychoactive substances, meaning they affect the receptors in the brain. They can cause euphoria, changes in consciousness, and distorted and/or enhanced perception. They are not entirely addictive (some are even non-addictive). However, their pleasant and rewarding effects to the mind are what draw people to continually seek them. For the sake of clarity, addiction is defined as the compulsive and continual use of a substance despite the detrimental effects.

Interestingly, most hallucinogens are derived from compounds found in plants and fungi. The active substances in such drugs have chemical structures that are similar to the brain's neurotransmitters.

Hallucinogens are not entirely illegal. A handful of them are used medically as anesthetics, anticonvulsants and for the treatment of ADHD, anxiety disorders, depression, sleep disorders and various neurological disorders. Some hallucinogens are even used to treat addiction to certain pharmaceutical and psychoactive drugs.

Hallucinogens can be classified into three main groups: psychedelics, dissociatives and deliriants. Despite the restrictions on hallucinogens, their usage is quite common in most countries as recreational drugs.

Psychedelics

The term "psychedelic" is derived from two Greek words that mean *to reveal* or *manifest the mind*. Examples of psychedelics include ayahuasca, LSD, Peyote, Psilocybin (aka magic mushrooms), morning glory seeds (ololiuqui), Harmine, 2C-1, methoxetamine, DMT and other tryptamine and phenethylamine drugs.

A type of marijuana called Sativa, or *Cannabis sativa*, is also a mild hallucinogen. Some psychedelics are synthetic while others are derived from natural sources, such as seeds, fungi, and leaves. Psychedelics cause alterations in vision and perception, and it is usually used interchangeably with the term *hallucinogens*.

The job of the active substances of psychedelics is to bind themselves to certain receptors (mainly serotonin receptors) in the brain and to interfere with neurotransmitters. Once they are bound to the receptors, the hallucinogenic effects take place, which varies depending on the active substances of the hallucinogen.

The hallucinogen would replace serotonin in these receptors. Their effects are prominent in the prefrontal cortex, the area of the brain behind your forehead, which processes emotion, mood, cognition and sensory perception. When used moderately, psychedelics are rarely intoxicating.

The effects of psychedelics are not limited to visual and auditory stimulation and relaxation. Emotions are almost always magnified once the active compounds bind to the receptors. Every bit of pleasant and unpleasant emotions is magnified profoundly, so this may subject users to panic attacks.

Users also become extremely sensitive to their environment, so every gesture and every movement around them seems surreal. It is also common that long forgotten memories and events from the distant past are "resurrected" or remembered. If someone has strived to forget a certain traumatic experience without proper closure, then psychedelics can make that person relive the traumatic event all over again.

Other typical sensations when consuming psychedelics include the following:

Feelings that all of the shallow worldly wants (money, fame, material gains, etc.) are meaningless or irrelevant

Loss of sense of time

Senses seem to have no boundaries

Mixed feelings of bliss, ecstasy, and anguish

Despite the generalities regarding the effects of psychedelics, some people have problems experiencing profound effects. The actual effects vary from person to person, and they depend on the circumstances that a user is in while tripping.

Dissociatives

The term "dissociatives" refers to the fact that the drugs under this classification are able to induce a feeling of detachment from their surroundings. They are classified as hallucinogens because they distort or alter a person's sense of reality and time. These substances cause a person to feel as if the events around him or her are fantasies or dreams (derealization).

In addition to this, dissociatives also induce a feeling of depersonalization. In this state, users feel as though they are not contained within their own physical bodies. They can see themselves, particularly their extremities (arms, legs, fingers, toes), but they fail in controlling their own movements. They also have a difficulty in recognizing themselves in the mirror. They feel as if they are watching themselves from a distance. In some cases, dissociative drugs induce out of body experiences.

Dissociative drugs work by blocking NMDA receptors all over the brain. When this happens, the neurotransmitter glutamate fails to exhibit its so-called life preserving effects, such as perception of pain, memory, and cognition. This leads to the senses being slightly dysfunctional. Some side effects include a rise or drop in respiration or heart rate.

Common dissociative drugs include nitrous oxide, DXM, MSE, PCP, ketamine (K, cat Valium), and diviner's sage (Salvia *divinorum*).

Side effects that are associated with dissociative drug abuse and misuse include memory loss, muscle numbness, tremors, anxiety, and impaired physical functions. Slight dizziness, numbness, and increased body temperature are normal. For high dosages, paranoia, panic, and feelings of invincibility can set in. Death can occur either by heart attack or by partaking in a dangerous physical stunt while under the influence of a dissociative.

Deliriants

Deliriants are substances that subject the user to a state of delirium and confusion. Users often lose the ability to control their motor movements. Most kinds of deliriants are sourced from plants such as henbane, deadly nightshade, mandrake, and nutmeg. Tobacco can also be a deliriant in high doses.

Deliriants may offer dark hallucinations, and in some cases, users may feel like they are being watched by something they don't know. Deliriants can also potentially cause aggression and rage.

Other Natural Sources of Hallucinogens

Nature is abundant in flora and fauna containing hallucinogenic substances. Here is a list of plants and fungi and the corresponding psychoactive substances they contain. A quick word of caution: this does not imply that you should venture out in search for that certain plant or mushroom. Remember that hallucinogenic substances need to be isolated, extracted, or purified first in some cases.

Mescaline
Peyote, Peruvian Torch Cactus, Bolivian torch cactus, San Pedro Cactus

DMT
Chaliponga, Chacruna, Jurema, Yopo, Vilca, Virola

THC and cannabinoids
Cannabis plant species

Ibogaine
Iboga

Tropane alkaloids
Jimson weed, Henbane

Harmala alkaloids
Ayahuasca, Harmal, Jurema, Mapacho,

Ergoline alkaloids
Christmas vine, Morning Glory, Hawaiian woodrose

Psilocybin, Baeocystin
Magic Mushroom species

Brief History

The consumption of hallucinogens by humans is not new. Archaeologists have discovered huffing bowls and crude pipes that are at least 2,000 years old with traces of hallucinogenic substances. This led to the conclusion that human ancestors used hallucinogenic substances, particularly for spiritual purposes.

Cave paintings and murals that show people taking (smoking, snorting, ingesting, etc.) organic hallucinogens reinforce this idea. Hallucinogens were (and still are by some) thought to establish a connection between the mortal (who is under the influence of the substance) and "the Divine," or other spiritual beings that belong to higher planes of consciousness. It was thus used before as an aid for transcendence during meditation and rituals.

Chapter 2:

Modern Developments

Hallucinogens are gradually and continually being studied for their medical applications. In fact, scientists have been studying and testing the potential of hallucinogens since the 1970's. They are specifically being explored as potential treatments for alcoholism, depression, nausea, and addiction to certain drugs such as opium. Because of their ability to distort perception, they are also being studied as a potential cure for bipolar disorder, schizophrenia, dementia and obsessive-compulsive disorder.

Scientists and doctors also tap on the potential of hallucinogens as an aid for terminally ill patients to alleviate their psychological angst and fear of death during the last days of their lives. LSD and psilocybin, for example, are being studied as a means for terminally ill patients to release their accumulated negative emotions, expand their perspective on life and death, and gain a more positive outlook in regards to letting go.

Recreational users of hallucinogens often wonder why the experiences can't also apply to healthy people. Serious problems often arise if healthy people take hallucinogens without proper guidance, which can lead them to a wide range of physiological and/or mental issues.

Doctors admit that hallucinogens have powerful and almost always positive effects (in proper dosages) on perception and consciousness. Researchers who explore the future medical applications for hallucinogens, particularly psilocybin and LSD, also speculate that hallucinogens are usually non-toxic and non-addictive compared to other illegal drugs.

LSD is even used to treat alcohol addiction. However, they refuse to label them as safe because of the danger that comes to users when one thinks he or she can fly or when a user can't orient him or herself properly because they can't see or hear like they normally would. In addition, those with a family history of psychosis are not advised to take hallucinogens.

With the increasing recreational use of hallucinogens by the general public and the increasing stigma surrounding it, some people resort to designer drugs and the so-called "research chemicals" to thwart legal punishments. Designer drugs are substances (specifically analogs of a drug) that aim to imitate the effects of said drug. Research chemicals, on the other hand, are compounds that are supposed to be used for research and experiments but not for human consumption. Technically, designer drugs are not illegal. Some countries, however, have restrictions on research chemicals.

Hallucinogens in Popular Culture

Are these substances evil or good? Today, the term hallucinogen, or specifically psychedelics, has been given a bad reputation, mainly because of their side effects. In part of the campaign to lessen the use of hallucinogens as substances used for fun and recreation, the people who become addicted to drugs in general are sensationalized in a negative way.

Hallucinogens, in general, are often demonized, but this doesn't mean that they are entirely detrimental to one's health. Likewise, hallucinogens are not entirely free from long-term side effects. People would no doubt inch themselves closer to death if they abuse them or took improper dosages and concoctions.

Hallucinogens are best viewed subjectively. They were used before as an aid in shamanistic rituals. This could indicate that hallucinogens occupy a rather respected reputation because they are associated with religious or spiritual journeys. One must wonder why they were so respected by our ancient ancestors. Maybe they understood just how much power and danger these intriguing substances possessed.

Chapter 3:

Overview of LSD, Peyote, Psilocybin and PCP

LSD

LSD stands for lysergic acid diethylamide, and it is colloquially called "acid." It is synthesized from ergotamine, a substance produced by a type of grain fungi. It used to be legally marketed as Delysid. The effects of a good and bad trip stay in one's memory. LSD is highly sensitive to UV light and oxygen, so exposing it to air and light can weaken or destroy it.

Pure LSD is odorless, colorless, and tasteless. It is however very potent - three pounds of LSD can provide equal effects to millions of people. The CIA even (unsuccessfully) tested the potential of LSD as a mind control agent for chemical warfare. About 20 to 30 micrograms is considered to be the threshold dose. Modes of administration include oral, intravenous, intramuscular, and sublingual (under the tongue).

Sublingual LSD is taken with gelatin sheets or square blotter paper sheets.

Effects

LSD causes long trips (up to 8 to 12 hours). The most noticeable effects of a good trip are an altered and expanded consciousness, in which the boundaries set by one's auditory, sensory, and visual senses are melted away, sounds seeming louder and richer, colors seeming more vibrant, surfaces appearing to glimmer, shine and ripple, emotions seeming to be more profound and your mental processes becoming more complex.

Additionally, objects seem to morph and random geometric shapes "scatter and crawl." Visual hallucinations can occur with closed or open eyes. Certain dosages can cause users to think more, leading to a rush of information and faster cognitive processing. Sometimes, synesthesia sets in. Tolerance builds up with constant use.

Normally, it takes around 20 to 120 minutes for the effects to be initially felt. The peak effects usually take place after 45 minutes. The body's temperature will rise, the pupils will dilate, and profuse sweating and nausea become common. A tingly sensation all over one's body may be felt. Taking LSD on an empty stomach or two hours after eating lessens nausea.

Once users hit the peak effects, the sensations can last around 2 to 5 hours. This is the times where hallucinations, flashbacks, and rush of emotions take place, and all of the sensations will feel real. Take note that delusion is also common at this stage, especially if one is not accompanied by at least one sober individual.

After Effects

The effects will usually start to wear down at around eight hours. However, users may feel tender and still quite disoriented until they get some sleep. Upon waking up, it is normal to feel drained and tired. A good trip will somehow give users a sense of blithe that can last for several days. Regular users of LSD also experience flashbacks (flashes of vivid colors, light, and hallucinations) long after taking the drug. Flashbacks are random and can occur anytime, anywhere.

Peyote

Peyote is a type of cactus. Its hallucinogenic abilities are attributed to the chemical called mescaline, which is also present in other hallucinogenic cacti, such as the San Pedro cactus. Mescaline binds to serotonin receptors in the brain, resulting in vivid hallucinations. Ancient religious groups in Mexico have used peyote. Some states in the U.S., such as Arizona and Nevada, allow civilians to possess peyote as long as it is used for religious practices. The San Pedro cactus is believed to be a good substitute for peyote.

Effects

Peyote usually causes an altered state of perception of time and one's surroundings. Moods seem magnified and exaggerated. First timers feel a certain fear of losing control, which is normal with all hallucinogens. Side effects include profuse sweating, increased heart rate, nausea, and flushing.

After Effects

Flashbacks tend to occur after consuming peyote. Long-term effects are not well established at this point in time.

Psilocybin

Psilocybin is a type of compound that binds to the serotonin receptors of the brain. It is derived from about 200 species of mushrooms. However, the concentration of psilocybin varies from species to species. Collectively, they are called psilocybin mushrooms. Psilocybin can be taken in one of two ways: orally or intravenously.

The active compounds are housed in the caps and stems. Spores do not contain psychedelic compounds. Alfred Hoffman first purified it from the *Psilocybe mexicana* mushroom. It was Hoffman who also synthesized LSD in 1938. Only an expert should source psilocybin because it is easy to mistake them for poisonous mushrooms.

Once psilocybin is metabolized in the body, it is converted to psilocin, to which euphoria and perception-altering properties are attributed. This substance is currently being studied for its effects against anxiety and depression. The legality of psilocybin varies. In the United Kingdom, for example, fresh psilocybin mushrooms are legal. In the United States, it is classified as a Schedule 1 drug (drugs with "no known medical use") with LSD and heroin.

Effects

Not only can it cause hallucinations but psilocybin can also cause synesthesia, which is the combination of two sensory functions. People under the influence of psilocybin can experience tasting or hearing colors. Synesthesia is also a neurological condition in which people claim to associate letters and sounds with colors.

Even if the hallucinogenic effects have waned, psilocybin makes an individual more open or receptive to new ideas. Just like Peyote, it is believed that humans before written history consumed psilocybin. Hallucinations can also occur even if one's eyes are closed, though hallucinations with psilocybin are very rarely confused with reality. Depersonalization does occur with psilocybin.

Unlike other hallucinogens, once psilocybin binds to the receptors in the brain, it exhibits a calming activity, rather than a stimulating one. Psilocybin thus removes the unnecessary "noises" and thoughts among adults.

Novices or first timers often experience panic attacks once the hallucinogenic effects of psilocybin take place. However, this substance has a low toxicity and cases of death are very rare. The body quickly adapts to psilocybin because it induces relaxing feelings. However, users are advised to take a 1 to 4 month break between psilocybin trips to avoid unpleasant after effects. The peak lasts for about 1 to 2 hours, depending on the strength of the dosage. A dosage of 2 grams (dried) or 20 grams (fresh) is considered reasonable for most people.

After Effects

If psilocybin trips are spaced appropriately, then negative after effects, such as psychological and nervous breakdowns, are rare. Proper dosages give users a certain feeling of "glow" that can linger for up to two months. Side effects of psilocybin include difficulty to concentrate flushing, profuse sweating, lightheadedness, dizziness, numbness, stomach pain, and frequent yawning.

PCP

PCP (phencyclidine) is a sedative narcotic commonly known as "rocket fuel," "angel's dust," "hog," "superweed," "ozone" or "wet." This substance prevents the neurotransmitter glutamase from binding to its receptors. PCP has no known medical use, although it was used briefly in the 1950's as an anesthetic.

It was phased out in 1965 for its side effects, but it is continually produced today in underground laboratories. PCP is quickly dissolved in alcohol or water. It is also available in tablet form. Aside from ingestion, it can also be snorted or injected. Some people sprinkle "angel's dust" to tobacco and marijuana joints. Oil-based PCP may be used as a dip for cigarettes and joints as well.

Effects

The effects of PCP take place in unpredictable periods. Taking this drug gives feelings of heightened euphoria and a sense of invincibility, which can lead to destructive behavior, such as leaping out of windows, self mutilation, or jumping in front of moving cars.

This is worsened by the fact that it drastically lessens the sensation to pain. At high dosages, it is believed to imitate schizophrenia. In addition to feeling high and intoxicated, a user's eyes will appear red, speech will be slurred, and balance cannot be maintained while walking. Some individuals experience cold sweating, vomiting and dizziness.

Needless to say, PCP is a very unreliable drug, as a dosage that is safe for one person may be lethal for another. Furthermore, dosages are hard to control since PCP has become more commonly available in powder form. Overdose can lead to a heart attack, coma, or even death. The substance remains traceable in the system for up to 30 days.

After Effects

The effects of PCP will wane after an indefinite number of hours because it is an unpredictable substance.

Health Risks of Hallucinogens

Hallucinogens are beneficial to some degree, but there are also numerous health risks. Unlike prescription drugs, it can be difficult to measure the proper dosage of hallucinogens. Moreover, people develop a degree of drug tolerance if they take it regularly.

This leads to the need to "up" the dosage, which can spiral into stronger tolerance and eventually overdosing. PCP, for example, is a hallucinogen that is highly unstable. As mentioned before, its effects vary from person to person. It should be noted that, even with proper guidance, PCP packs a greater risk compared to other hallucinogens.

Short-term side effects will wane, but long-term side effects are usually permanent or require therapy or professional treatment to be cured. The health risks depend on the amount taken, the frequency of dosage, and the current health history of the user. Family history of mental illnesses increases the risk of negatively reacting to hallucinogens.

Pregnant and breast-feeding women should avoid taking hallucinogens. PCP, among others, has the ability to cross the placental barrier. Although there are not many substantial studies that cement the negative effects of hallucinogens to pregnant and breast-feeding women, it remains clear that the unborn fetus and babies are harmed because their brains are not yet fully developed. The interactions of hallucinogens with prescription medications are also not fully understood at this point.

Costs

How much do hallucinogens cost? Why and how can young teenagers afford them? Hallucinogens do not come with a suggested retail price, nor are their prices regulated. Nevertheless, hallucinogens are not entirely affordable. LSD costs about $10 for more or less a 75-microgram hit. Take note of the phrase "more or less." This means that the exact amount of LSD is not precisely determined. You could be taking *more* or *less* than 75 micrograms.

Magic mushrooms are available in fresh and dried variants. It can cost about $25 for 35 grams of fresh magic mushrooms and about 3 grams of the dried variant mushrooms. Additionally, the price may vary depending on the mushroom species because some mushrooms contain higher concentrations of psilocybin. Peyote costs about $5 to $8 per button, and about 10 buttons are needed for the effects to be felt. An ounce of liquid PCP costs about $125 to $600.

Chapter 4:

Pros and Cons

Pros

Popular hallucinogens, such as LSD and psilocybin, are not addictive because they are purely psychedelic, unlike empathogen and entactogen drugs, such as ecstasy, MDMA, and MDEA. However, if a person craves the feelings of escapism, then they have the potential to be dependent on LSD and psilocybin.

Some hallucinogens have the potential to curb addiction. Psilocybin, for example, can help cigarette-addicted patients quit smoking. A study conducted at John Hopkins University School of Medicine tested the efficiency of psilocybin to nicotine addiction, and all test subjects quit smoking. A year later, all but one of them had abstained from smoking since their first session with psilocybin.

Cons

Some hallucinogenics can cause a bad trip. LSD, for example, undergoes a careful synthesis, and if you got a low quality product, then the effects can leave you traumatized for the same length of time that the desirable effects take place. Some first timers panic once the effects of the hallucinogenic set in. Unfortunately, they rarely can control their panic. There are a lot of instances in which people (especially teenagers) run into highways and jump off balconies and overpasses out of sheer panic.

To avoid this, a trusted sober person, who has also taken the drug before, should accompany first timers. Panic attacks are common, but it can be alleviated by verbal assurances, comforting and protective acts, such as hugging and caressing. In some cases, some people experience acute psychotic reactions that last more than 24 hours, leading to hospitalization.

Short-Term and Long-Term Effects

Just like most substances, hallucinogenics have unpleasant side effects. Long-term use may promote feelings of psychological dependence. Long-term users may also begin to consistently search for the pleasant sensations brought about by hallucinogens. Once dependence sets in, a person will need to undergo drug rehabilitation to end the cycle.

Short-term effects depend on the substance taken. Usually, these are brief but substantial physical occurrences, such as shortness of breath, redness of the eyes, sleeplessness, and loss or increase of appetite. Most users equate the intense euphoria and bliss to enlightenment. The mind can't seem to stay on one mood, thought, or idea. Some users feel as if their bodies are liquefying, expanding, or dissipating, as if they are no longer physically present. Some other possible short-term effects include the following:

Dizziness, nausea and trembling

Numbness and muscle cramps

Dry mouth

Profuse sweating and chills (cold sweating)

Goose bumps

Poor coordination and difficulty in walking

High body temperature (mescaline, peyote) or low body temperature (LSD, psilocybin)

Faster heart rate (LSD, psilocybin) or depressed heart rate (mescaline, peyote)

Seizures

Slurred speech and drooling (PCP)

Rapid eye movements and blurred visions (PCP)

Suicidal thoughts connected to assumptions of being invincible (PCP)

PCP can also provide side effects such as paranoia, irrational behavior, and violent outbursts. Long-term usage can lead to an increased heart rate and blood pressure. Because of its unreliable nature, the short and long-term side effects, such as hallucination, paranoia, slurred speech, and fast respiration, vary for each individual.

With long-term use, users can experience erratic mood swings. Here is a list of more possible long-term effects of hallucinogens:

Physical and psychological dependence (leading to anxiety and depression if a person misses a dosage)

Tolerance (leading the user to up his or her dosage to feel the desired effects)

Liver damage

Flashbacks

Birth defects and miscarriages

Memory loss and impaired cognitive ability (PCP)

Permanent difficulty in speech (PCP)

Excessive weight loss (PCP)

When it comes to the skin, high dosages of hallucinogens can cause dry skin. The active chemicals affect the central nervous system, so manifestations such as skin lesions, itches, and gray lips are non-evident, unless they are mixed with other drugs that cause such.

Final Word

Some people resort to drugs, and hallucinogens in particular, in order to find a meaningful path in life, and others use them to self-medicate anxiety disorders and depression. Without proper guidance, many people end up addicted or turned off to the sensations and trip brought about by hallucinogenics.

The active compounds can lift you up to heights you never imagined seeing, but sooner or later one has to learn to come back to the ground and face life's challenges. There is nothing wrong (at least not in the eyes of the law) about exploring your spirituality and senses with hallucinogens. It is true that most aspects of human beings are masked by a false sense of happiness.

With moderate use *and* proper guidance, hallucinogens can help you live life to the fullest, but they should not be shortcuts or substitutes for anything. A lot of people, especially teenagers, fall into false and romanticized claims about hallucinogens (i.e. it will make you feel enlightened, you will experience heaven and hell at once, etc.) in general without regard that there are different types of hallucinogens that will react differently to each person's body chemistry.

If you decide to consume hallucinogens, then make sure to start with the lowest dosage. Space your "sessions" accordingly to avoid bad after effects and to decrease your body's tolerance to the hallucinogen.

You are paying a very big price if you want to take hallucinogens to mimic celebrities or to appear cool and sophisticated. Likewise, mixing hallucinogens with other drugs, without sufficient knowledge about their combined effects, may cause irreversible damage or even death.

If you find yourself gradually becoming addicted to hallucinogens, then seek help immediately. A quick online search regarding drug rehabilitation hotlines will yield several helpful rehabilitation centers that will help you break the cycle. Curiosity is normal, but when it comes to drugs pair it with responsibility and proper guidance from someone who has experience and a sound judgment (not someone who is trying to upsell you drugs). Finally, be mentally prepared and strong because bad trips are not unusual.

Chapter 5:

Hallucinogens vs. Other Drugs

How do Hallucinogens Compare to Other Drugs?

Hallucinogens appeal to most people because of the vivid visual and auditory trips and distorted perception of time they offer. Certain hallucinogens are not addictive. However, some people still develop dependence because they crave the blissful feelings hallucinogens offer. Just like other drugs, hallucinogens have the potential to induce tolerance that drives the user to increase his or her dosage. Hallucinogens also carry risks identical with other kinds of drugs.

Facts and Trivia About Hallucinogens

Now that you have a brief but substantial background of hallucinogens, it is time to explore more facts regarding them. Textbook knowledge about these substances is always helpful, but it is better if you have miscellaneous knowledge about them.

DMT, a substance considered to be a psychedelic, naturally occurs in the body. The pituitary gland secretes high amounts of DMT during the infancy stage, orgasms, and when a person is about to die. Scientists speculate that the intense rush of DMT in the brain cause near-death experiences (NDE), in which a person sees a tunnel of light and spiritual guides/angels. Just like DMT, cannabis has chemicals that also occur endogenously.

The discovery of the hallucinogenic effects of LSD was not intentional. It was synthesized on November 16th, 1938, but it was not until five years later that Hoffman experienced his first *trip*. At first he panicked, but later he purposely took LSD to verify its effects. It was during a bicycle ride home that he felt the effects of LSD, thus Bicycle Day was born. Hoffman even admitted to liking the effects of LSD.

Humans do not own the domain of hallucinogens. Animals take hallucinogens on purpose, too. Horses, bighorn sheep, and reindeers are the most common animals to get trippy. Their favorite substances are locoweed, lichens, and magic mushrooms. Somehow they know which mushrooms are poisonous and which are safe for consumption. Dogs also lick a species of toad to get trippy on the natural hallucinogenic substances found on the toads' skin.

Bees also experience a powerful trip (voluntarily or involuntarily) when they collect nectars of hallucinogenic plants. Birds deliberately eat marijuana seeds and peck on marijuana buds to get high. Other animals that consume psychoactive substances include rats, lizards, spiders, and mice. Some do it for fun whereas others, particularly those from the male species, do it before picking a fight against other male species to win a potential mate.

Some people get high on animal urine. Yes, that's right. Animals, particularly reindeers that consume magic mushrooms, still have the active hallucinogenic substances in their urine. There is an Alaskan tribe that collects and drinks the urine of reindeers to get high.

There is an ongoing debate as to whether hallucinogens help people achieve an altered state of consciousness in which they are able to tune in to extraterrestrial forces and means of communication. The currently accepted consensus about hallucinogens, particularly psychedelics, is that they affect the body's senses, leading to a seemingly real interaction with one's imagination. However, there are speculations that psychedelics, specifically DMT, open up the "channel" in the human mind that makes communication possible with beings belonging to other planes of consciousness.

LSD is the most abused and misused psychedelic. It is highly available, yet extremely powerful. Pregnant women who consume LSD during the pregnancy often give birth to babies with physical defects.

Conclusion

Thank you for reading this! We hope this short, concise book was able to teach you a thing or two about hallucinogens.

Now that you understand the important factors regarding hallucinogens, you can decide if you want to try them, or if you can inform your friends who ask you about the topic. Plus, a little addition to your knowledge doesn't hurt, right? Our world is becoming increasingly interested in the use of hallucinogenic substances, in hopes to enhance the human experience on Earth.

If you've learned anything from this book, please take the time to share your thoughts by sending me a personal message, or even posting a review on Amazon. It would be greatly appreciated and I try my best to get back to every message!

Thank you and good luck on your journey!

Printed in Great Britain
by Amazon